Are You Eating to Live While Dieting And Losing Weight?

M. Johnson

ISBN-10: 1468023543
ISBN-13: 978-1468023541

DEDICATION

This book is dedicated to all who are struggling with weight management and also those who are discouraged and don't think that they will ever accomplish their goal.

Introduction

Do you hesitate to start losing weight because you don't know what foods are effective in helping you to lose those extra pounds? You may want to get started but you also want to eat to live while you're losing weight.

Losing weight should never be an unpleasant task. Eating the right foods while dieting should be a pleasant adventure and not a dreary task; however, without the right foods and instructions, you may not be successful.

Learn how to motivate yourself to lose weight, learn what foods to eat while dieting. Also learn what foods not to eat while dieting.

Dieting and exercise have great benefits and should be included for your weight loss success. Take charge of successfully getting in good shape for better health.

You will find in this book information to help you accomplish your weight loss goal.

Introduction

3 THINGS TO KNOW BEFORE DIETING

1. Why Do You Want To Diet? The answer to this question is not necessarily obvious. People have many different reasons to diet. Surprising, all reasons are not about being overweight. You must first identify why you want to diet. This is very important to know because it allows you to analyze where you are and where you want to be. Identifying the purpose will also keep you focused on your goal.

2. Set Attainable Goals. Perhaps the reason why you were on the stop and go merry-go-round is because you had the desire to start a dieting program, however you did not set any goals or any attainable goals to help you accomplish your desire.

Now, lets say that you wanted to shed about 10 lbs. How would you do so? Would you stop eating junk foods, would you stop eating carbs, would you eliminate sweets or would you just reduce the number of meals you eat per day? Keep in mind that all carbs aren't bad and all sweets aren't detrimental.

Dieting is easier when you have a plan. Not only should you set attainable goals but you should also commit to following them.

3. Educate Yourself.

Take time to learn how to maintain your goal once you've reached it. This is one of the main reasons why so many people find themselves starting and stopping a weight loss program. They begin feeling defeated and discouraged and allow their feelings to stop them from making the desired change that they want.

3 WAYS TO LOSE WEIGHT WITHOUT DIETING

First Suggestion:

Walking consistently. Anytime I begin to notice extra pounds, one of the first things that I do is to start walking. Walking is one of the best ways for me to drop some extra pounds because I burn calories when I consistently walk. I prefer walking in the evenings because it allows me time to relieve any stress I encountered during the day.

Sometimes I speed walk and then at other times I walk a longer distance however, there is no set pattern to my choice. The method I use is based on how I may be feeling at the time. There are times that I just don't feel like walking at a constant fast pace, therefore I don't. The key factor for me is just simply to walk frequently.

The other reason I like to walk in the evening is because I have the opportunity to burn my evening meal calories. You know, the slice of apple pie and perhaps the ice cream. Sometimes I just like clearing my mind and thinking about my goals such as losing some pounds. I feel so much refreshed after I've been walking. It makes me feel positive.

Second Suggestion:

Eat breakfast and don't eat late in the evening. When you start your day with a full stomach you're less likely to snack throughout the day. You're less likely to get hungry. Also eat more fruits and vegetables they will provide you with fiber and also can be quite filling. Add protein to your meals because it will help keep you feeling full. A cup of grapes as a snack can replace the candy bar you may be accustomed to having.

Third Suggestion:

Drink a lot of water. Water has so many benefits besides being an important aid to losing weight. Water flushes toxins from your system as well as fight fatigue. Drink it throughout the day. Water is also good for your skin and muscle tone; don't allow yourself to become dehydrated. Water also makes your metabolism burn calories faster. I bet now you appreciate water a little more don't you?

Well, I hope these 3 suggestions helps you as they have helped me. In addition to me implementing these 3 things I also make sure I watch what and how I eat.

1 REASON WHY WEIGHT LOSS CAN BE EASY

The key to the effects of the outcome that you encounter in life is linked to your thoughts. Your thoughts hold much power that you may not be aware of. Have you ever noticed that when you are experiencing something unpleasant, you can think about something that is pleasant and then you begin to feel better?

Imagine not feeling well and you decide to stay at home for the day. Now, since you may be an active person who is always on the go, having to stay at home may be quite difficult for you. However, you take advantage of the inconvenience of being home bound. You may begin to imagine being on an island where you can have your favorite meals and beverages, while laying in a gently swinging hammock that's near the cool waters.

Imagine being on a shopping spree that you've just won and there is no limitation of how many purchases you can put in you cart. How does that thought make you feel? Doesn't the thought of that make you feel better?

Well, the reason why losing weight can be made easy is because of your thoughts. Even though losing weight has its challenges, the way that you approach it determines the effects of its outcome.

Here are 3 tips to help make losing weight easy:

-Eat low calorie and low fat foods that you like.
-Wear attractive workout clothes while you're exercising.
-Keep positive thoughts about the outcome.

Remember to take control of your thoughts.
If you think positively you will have a positive attitude, which will give you positive weight loss results. Imagine yourself reaching those goals.

HOW TO BE POSITIVE ABOUT WEIGHT LOSS - 3 TIPS

1. Positive Thoughts Result In Positive Outcome.

Some people don't succeed at weight loss because of their negative thoughts. Instead of focusing on the difficult things, you should focus on the things that you do well. Positive thinking motivates you into doing things that would even surprise yourself.

You should make a game out of weight loss. Create your own personal game that will keep losing weight fun and not boring.

Don't look down on yourself. (Especially don't let others look down on you). You can't really change how others perceive you.

2. Keep in mind that you are unique.

Your situation is not like others therefore you should design a plan that you're comfortable with. You may have a friend that is also fighting the weight loss battle, so therefore try teaming up together and you will always have something to talk about and to share your ups and downs with concerning weight loss.

Choose a favorite weight loss book. This is something that you can keep handy and read anytime you're needing encouragement. Don't get discouraged to the point of quitting. Anytime that you are feeling overwhelmed, that is the time to take a break.

3. Remember to pace yourself.

Don't be in such a hurry that you get exhausted. You didn't put the weight on over night; therefore allow yourself the proper amount of time to drop the extra weight. If you maintain a positive attitude through you weight loss venture, you will be surprised at the positive outcome.

5 THINGS TO DO WHILE LOSING WEIGHT

Don't allow your feelings to alter you weight loss plans. You should create a plan that is flexible for those days that you may not feel well. Don't allow feelings to stop you from reaching your weight loss goals. Be determined to meet your needs. Five things you should do while losing weight are:

1. Monitor Your Caloric Intake.

You must educate yourself about the foods you eat. Some things that you may think don't have many calories may be the very things that are hindering your weight loss progress. Begin by reading the ingredients label. Watch your portions. Just because something maybe low in calories doesn't mean that you should eat extremely large portions. Remember to do the math. A small amount of anything multiplied by a large amount equals a large amount.

2. Drink Plenty of Water.

Sufficient water intake is essential to your overall health. One of the benefits of water is that it eliminates fatigue. Fatigue is one of the main reasons why some people stop with their weight loss program. Also get use to drinking a glass of water before you eat because it will give you a feeling of being full. When you feel full you eat less.

3. Get Sufficient Rest.

When you're rested you make better decisions. Resting reserves energy to exercise and to think clearly. Remember that your thoughts determine your destiny.

4. Eat Fruits and Vegetables.

Your body typically craves what it is accustomed to taking in. If you eat fruits & vegetables this is what your body will tell you that it wants and needs. For example try snacking on grapes instead of candy. Snacking on grapes can make you feel full and because of the water content you will be providing your body with the water it needs.

5. Be Positive

You should be your biggest fan. Learn how to encourage yourself and don't rely on others to comment. Follow your plan and then commend yourself for being committed to it.

KEYS TO FAT BURNING
SUCCESS ARE INGREDIENTS

Protein- Eating more protein burns calories and helps you to become lean. It's important to keep your protein intake high when dieting to make sure that you don't burn off any muscle tissue.

Foods that are high in protein and fiber are the best kinds of food to eat if you want to burn fat around your middle. In order to burn fat, you must eat frequently and not starve yourself

You should eat 5 or 6 times a day. Several smaller meals a day speeds up your metabolism and a high-speed metabolism is the secret to weight and fat loss.

A diet rich in lean protein can raise your RMR (Resting Metabolic Rate) by as much as 68%.

So just by eating protein, you immediately speed up your metabolic fire, thereby enabling your body to increase lean muscle mass and decrease body fat faster.

The average person typically needs 0.8-1 grams of protein per 1 kg of body weight to sustain a healthy muscle mass and overall good health.

Physical activity, illnesses, or taking certain medication may change your need for protein.

Proteins introduce fewer calories into your body's system than fat or carbohydrates. A diet rich in proteins, along with regular strength or resistance training, works to maintain or increase a body's lean muscle mass.

Peanut butter has important qualities, which makes it an ideal snack if you are trying to lose weight. In addition to its protein, fiber and healthy fat content, peanut butter also contains more than 30 essential vitamins and minerals. These include niacin, folate, potassium and vitamin E. Niacin is a B vitamin that helps convert food into energy. You can spread it on celery sticks, whole grain crackers, or apples.

Celery

Celery will fill you up and help expend even more calories in the fat-burning process. Celery has about 5 calories per serving, and your body probably burns about 5 to 10 calories digesting it. Eating celery will not burn enough calories to contribute to significant weight loss but on the other hand, if you just feel the need to munch on something while on a diet, celery is a great option because it won't really add calories.

Fruits and vegetables promote weight loss because they.

- Are very low in fat.
- Are low in calories.
- Are high in fiber, vitamins and minerals.
- Eliminate wastes quickly and help reduce cravings for sweets.
- Keep your energy levels steady so you don't become too hungry or too tired.
- Carry off excess body acids, and are rich in vitamins, minerals and enzymes that satisfy the body's nutrient requirements with less food.

10 FOODS TO EAT WHILE DIETING

You may have heard that carbohydrates are bad for you, however since you do need certain carbs, they are good and also bad. The good carbs are beneficial to us when it's full of fiber such as vegetables, fruits, beans and whole grains, which are filled with fiber and are beneficial to you..

Not only do good carbs have fiber but also they have vitamins and minerals. Now you may be thinking that fiber is not absorbable so how can it be good for you. Well, fiber does many good things for your body. It can definitely help with your weight management program. You should begin to read the food labels for fiber-enhanced foods.

If the fiber is soluble it moves bulk through the intestines and it promotes regular bowel movement and prevents constipation. It also assists in moving toxin waste from your colon and helps in keeping an optimal ph intestine, which can help with cancer prevention.

Dark leafy vegetables are a good source of insoluble fiber. The skins of fruits and vegetables are also good sources of insoluble fiber. How about whole-wheat products? It's a great source.

There is also soluble fiber, which binds with fatty acids and prolong stomach-emptying time so that sugar is released and absorbed slower. Soluble fiber also can lower your total cholesterol and regulate blood sugar.

Do you remember the saying "An apple a day keeps the doctor away"? Well one of the reasons that apples are extremely good for you is because of the fiber it has.

You may not think so but oranges also have fiber. Don't get confused about the types of fiber. The main thing to know is that fiber is good for you and many foods consist of both types. So just choose foods that have fiber in it and let your body reap the benefits.

Here is a list of 10 foods that you should eat while you're dieting:

- Salads- Be sure to include tomato, cabbage, lettuce or cucumber.

- Grapes- Eat a cup of grapes and see how full you feel. They're good for a snack.
- Potatoes- Yes, potatoes baked without the fatty additions.
- High Fiber Cereal- This can really full you up.
- Water- Drink a lot of water because it flushes your system and eliminate fatigue
- Beans- There are many to choose from
- Vegetables- You can even eat as snacks throughout the day
- Pasta- you can have it believe it or not.
- Crackers- make sure you read the label
- Whole grain breads- Imagine a tomato sandwich (yummy!)

Remember that in your quest to stick to a weight management program, food can be a help you when you make the right selections.

NUMBER 1 REASON WHY FIBER IS IMPORTANT FOR DIETS

Fiber is found in so many different kinds of food. There was a time prior to 1970s that we didn't hear much about fiber. I believe that if it was well known years ago many would not be dealing with sicknesses that they currently have. Your health should be the most important thing to you.

Imagine if you didn't have any fiber to consume. Not a pleasant thought is it? Fiber makes you feel full and for this reason it is an excellent weight loss aid. The one thing that you should make sure to do is drink a lot of water. When fiber intake is increased then water intake should be increased.

One of the many benefits of fiber is that it helps reduce the risk of some chronic diseases. On average North Americans consume less than 50 % of the dietary fiber levels recommended for good health.

You can get fiber from whole grains, beans, nuts, fruits and vegetables. Fiber should be added to your diet slowly because it can lead to excess gas and bloating. The amount of fiber you get everyday depends on your age and your sex.

Many people may not consume the recommended amounts in their foods therefore they would purchase supplements. Yet, there are others who do both.

The #1 reason why fiber is important for your diet is: It promotes overall health.

WAYS TO ENJOY YOUR FOOD AND LOSE WEIGHT

I've made the decision that I will not avoid the enjoyment of eating at a restaurant in fear of gaining a few extra pounds and or hindering my weight management progress.

I like writing while I'm enjoying a good meal. Even now as I write this article I'm sitting in a well-known 24-hour restaurant enjoying a mushroom & spinach omelet with 2 buttermilk pancakes. Yes, indeed it is delicious! You see delicious doesn't have to equate to fatty or greasy. If you're wondering how to enjoy your food and lose weight here are 4 ways.

1. Be Selective Choose low fat and low sugar foods. All delicious foods don't have to be high in calories and fat.

2. Eat Smaller Quantities. If you know that you may be eating something that is over your caloric limit, then eat a small portion but you have to be disciplined enough to do so.

3. Drink Plenty of Water. Drink a glass of water before you begin to eat. Water will give you a feeling of being full and you won't overeat. You will be able to eat and enjoy your food and you won't run the risk of overeating because you will feel full.

4. Exercise - Exercising will burn fat and calories. While you're exercising you'll also stimulate your mind and perhaps you won't feel to guilty about what you ate. Just walk an extra 1/2-mile.

Now the way to enjoy your food is to think about the goals you having met already! This will put you in a good mood and you will definitely enjoy your food.

Losing weight can be difficult without a guide and some instructions to help you with each step. Remember you can do this.

3 WAYS OF LOSING WEIGHT FAST

1. Determine how much weight you would like to lose.

A lot of times people who are pursuing a weight loss venture get frustrated simply because they don't have a plan. You should do an assessment to determine how much weight you want to lose and how you plan to lose it.

 When you don't assess your personal situation you will begin to do what everyone else is doing. One day you may be doing what you heard someone talking about until you hear about yet what someone else is doing and then you decide to switch to something else.

Do your assessment for your own personal venture based on what your needs is and what you will physically be able to follow through with. Seek your physician's advice because what you want to do may not be what you need to do.

Your weight loss venture should be pleasurable. If you are completely miserable because of what you are doing to achieve fast weight loss, then you should consider making changes to your weight loss plan. When you are mentally distressed over losing weight it will hinder your progress and you may even become discouraged and quit.

2. Exercise

Every weight loss program should include exercise. One of the key factors to weight loss is definitely exercise. Walking is very effective. You can do it on your break at work. You can even walk in place. The main thing is to just start walking. Walking will help you lose weight quickly because walking burns a lot of calories. You may incorporate other exercises that you are comfortable with doing.

3. Commitment

Regardless of which exercise program you start, unless you're committed you will not achieve your goal. Read positive information concerning the benefits of losing weight. When you begin to feel a little discourage, that's a good time to exercise to clear your mind. Remember that a lack of commitment slows the results.

3 TIPS FOR WOMEN TO LOSE BELLY FAT

Tip #1 - Ab Exercises

Exercise helps to burn extra calories and fat. It also tones the body so that you would be admirable in your new swimwear. Your exercise can be as simple as going for walks. As a matter of fact walking is one of the best exercises for burning fat. While you're walking why don't you think about what style of swimwear would look best on you.

Remember to consider the shape of your body so that you would not choose swimwear that won't compliment you.

Exercising would also relieve stress. Stress is the reason why some women over eat. It can cause slow digestion and anxiety. Also you should do some exercises that target your abdominal muscles. The lower abdomen is the most difficult area on the body to get firmed up. So pay close attention to your progress in this area. You will be happy when you start to see and feel the changes.

Tip#2 - Body Building Diets

Begin to eat to acquire lean muscle mass. Learn the role of carbohydrates, fats and proteins. Don't forget to monitor your caloric intake. Your diet and nutrition intake would play a very important part in how successful you are in losing your belly fat.

Vitamin and mineral intake is vital therefore don't neglect it. It you'd like you can use bodybuilding supplements to help with the fat burning process.

Tip#3 - Determination

Determination is the key to your success. Regardless of how things may appear at the time, don't give up. Sometimes a gradual change may be the best thing because it would allow your body time to adjust. Be consistent and maintain the new routine you have started. Before you know it you will have reached your goal.

3 REASONS WHY YOU SHOULD DETOX

You spend time cleaning up on the outside. However, have you stopped to think your inside needs to be cleaned also? What if you didn't ever take a shower or bath? What if you never used soap or a cleaning agent? Your body would accumulate layers and layers of dirt & debris. Begin to make your health the top priority in your life.

Here are three reasons why you should detox:

1. To Remove Excess Waste From You Digestive Tract.

Detoxing will rid your digestive tract of waste that has build up in your colon. It relieves you of bloating and your intestines become lighter in weight. You can eliminate harmful substances from your body that may be responsible for diseases and abnormalities.

2. To Lose Weight.

It helps you to get rid of unwanted pounds. Detox removes toxins this will cause your body to properly function resulting in your food being made to break down and eliminated. Losing weight would help you feel good, have more energy and reduce your risk for diseases.

3. To Increase Vitality and Energy Levels.

Are you always tired and just don't know why. It could be due to toxin build up from medications, foods and the environment. Imagine having a toxin build up for several years. This could be why you may continuously be tired. Detox provides a natural source of energy. Your mind will also be clearer and you may notice that you are more alert and focused.

WHAT YOU WANTED TO KNOW ABOUT VITAMINS

It is essential that we be aware of what constitutes good food health vitamin intake. The federal drug administration produces a recommended daily allowance for the majority of vitamins, which regards as a good food health vitamin intake.

We all should be aware that we do not get all of the vitamin and minerals that our bodies properly need. If a person is on a constrained diet for any reason then they need to pay even more attention to their good food health vitamin intake. Supplements should be used to supplement your diets and not replace it.

There are many different types of foods that we eat that help protect us. Our body can take the food that we eat and turn it into energy. However, our body can't produce all that we need in order to survive.

However, if you're not getting the vitamins and minerals that you need, you are going to find that your body is not functioning properly. This is why some people choose to use vitamin and mineral supplements because they know they aren't getting the proper amount of vitamins and minerals through what they eat.

Vitamin E is very important because without it, the cell membranes would be damaged. Which could lead to serious health problems, including cancer. Vitamin E is effective against free radicals because it is fat-soluble therefore it can be absorbed into the cell membranes. It is therefore essential for your immune system. A person's body weight determines the required amount.

VEGETARIAN'S HEALTHY CHOICE

Even though vegetarians eat a sufficient amount of protein, they don't take in as much as they frequently would on a non-vegetarian diet because plant proteins are considerably less digestible than animal proteins

Many begin without dedicating ample amount of time to research and meal planning. As a result, substantial amounts of people who start this type diet do not last longer than 1-2 months.

By eating vegetables, legumes, seeds, nuts, fruits, and whole grains, they can increase the amount of complete proteins they create by combining a number of varieties of amino acid chains.

They must eat a variety of plant proteins to form complete amino chains in order for them to absorb a healthy amount of protein. Also they have a number of options to boost their protein intake.

You should think about taking advantage of each option. You should expand your food selections, drink more soy products, and eat "protein-fortified" pasta and breads.

Usually you typically hear of adults changing to this type diet. Have you ever considered how many children change each year? It is possible to get your child to convert as well with a few tips in hand, it will be much easier than you may have thought. Choose what is best for you and your family. Healthy eating is very important.

It is going to take some effort to make the transition to a meatless lifestyle and to be able to say, "I am a vegetarian." But instead of feeling anxious by that prospect, make it a hobby also. Make it fun and enjoy the meatless eating experience.

Eventually, this exciting lifestyle will move from a passion to a hobby. It should be such an integral

part of your lifestyle. There is a lot of variety in a meatless lifestyle that will keep you fascinated for a long time.

FOOD EFFECTS BODY AND MIND

Food effects body and spirit and is very powerful. It can affect your mood and even how you think. Food can bring on all types of emotions. Try eating something you really like and watch how your mood changes. Food is so powerful that when you have a lack of food then you become hungry, then your mood changes. You may be grumpy, have shorter patient, irritable or even restless.

The Effects of Food on Your Body and Mind...

Is very crucial. Foods like turkey, snacks with sugar, and whole grain breads, raise and lower mood-altering chemicals, which affects the brain.

Food affects our lifestyle. The food choices we make will decide the outcome of our moods because food effects body and-mind. The average consumer unfortunately isn't eating a healthy enough diet, that will put them in a good mood."

A diet mistake that can lead to low moods is allowing your blood sugar to rise and fall through out the day. Then you may begin to crave foods that would raise your serotonin level. Serotonin is a neurotransmitter that is responsible for your moods, sleep and appetite. Remember that food effects body and spirit.

You may suffer from memory loss if you eat an unhealthy diet consisting of sugary carbohydrates. You may also feel depressed. You would also be likely to gain weight.

Do you see how important a healthy diet is to a hearty and healthy lifestyle? Food Effects Body and Spirit. Our diets cause us to function or not to function properly.

For more informational resources visit:

http://www.hearty-lifestyle-healthy-tips.com

http://www.webhealthmart4u.com

Have a Wonderful Day!

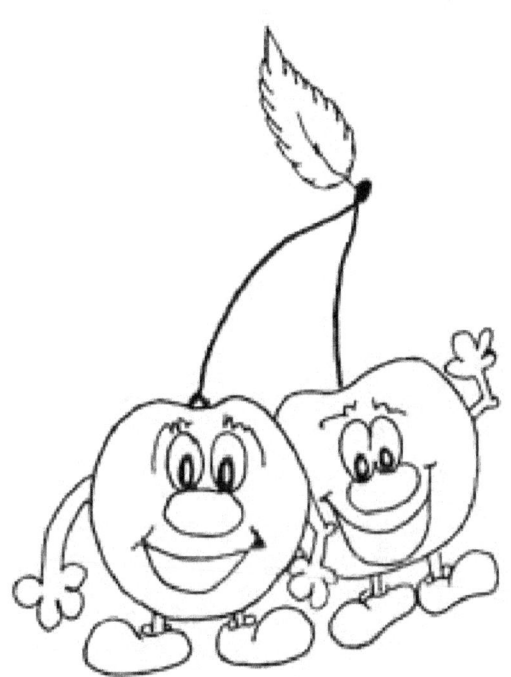